Kidney Dialysis

Diet Cookbook for Women Over 50

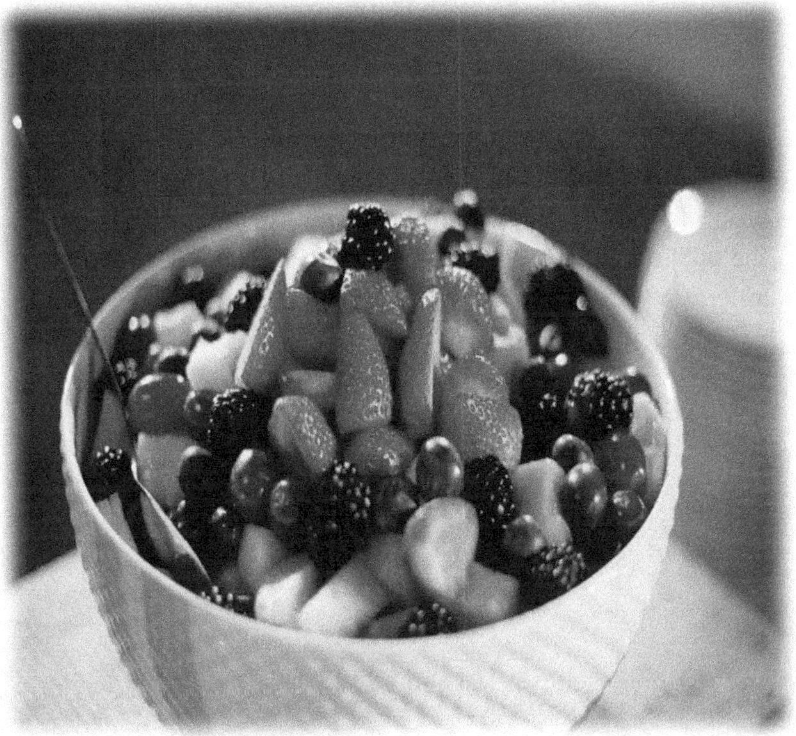

Hector A Anderson

Table of Contents

Thank you

I am writing to express my sincere gratitude for your interest in my book. Your decision to explore the pages of my work is not only deeply appreciated but also serves as a source of inspiration to me.

I look forward to hearing your thoughts by leaving a honest review on Amazon after exploring the various recipes and other insights in the book. Your feedback is very valuable to me and other authors like me

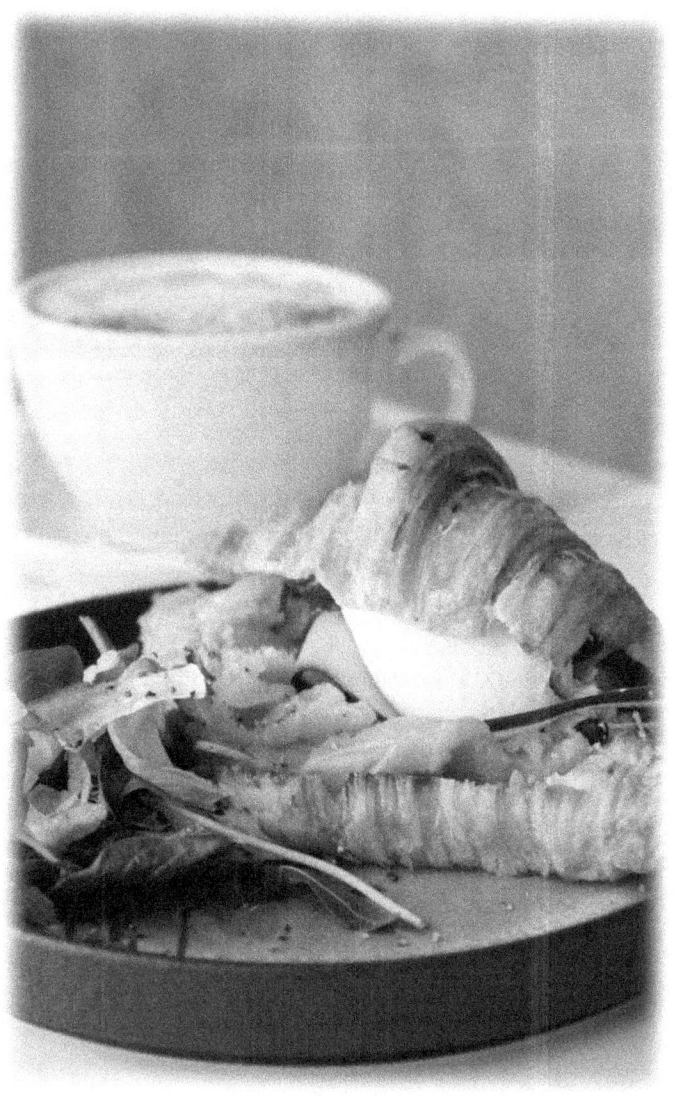

Introduction

Welcome to the beginning of your journey towards better kidney health and well-being through diet and nutrition. This chapter serves as your guide, providing essential information and support as you embark on this important path.

Understanding Kidney Disease and Dialysis

In this section, we delve into the fundamentals of kidney disease and the role of dialysis in managing its symptoms and complications. Understanding the basics of your condition is crucial for making informed decisions about your diet and lifestyle.

1. What is Kidney Disease?

Explanation of kidney function and the role of kidneys in maintaining overall health.

Common causes and risk factors for kidney disease, including diabetes, hypertension, and aging.

Stages of kidney disease and how they affect kidney function.

2. Introduction to Dialysis

Explanation of dialysis and its role in managing kidney failure.

Types of dialysis: hemodialysis and peritoneal dialysis.

Frequency and duration of dialysis sessions.

3. Symptoms and Complications of Kidney Disease

Common symptoms experienced by individuals with kidney disease, such as fatigue, fluid retention, and electrolyte imbalances.

Complications of kidney disease, including anemia, bone disease, and cardiovascular issues.

4. Impact of Diet on Kidney Health

Overview of the importance of diet in managing kidney disease.

How certain nutrients and dietary factors can affect kidney function.

The role of a specialized kidney dialysis diet in improving outcomes and quality of life.

5. Working with Your Healthcare Team

Importance of communication with your healthcare providers, including nephrologists, dietitians, and other specialists.

How to actively participate in your treatment plan and advocate for your needs.

Building a supportive network of family, friends, and community resources.

By gaining a deeper understanding of kidney disease and dialysis, you empower yourself to take control of your health and make informed choices that will support your journey towards improved well-being. Remember, you are not alone in this journey, and with the right knowledge and support, you can thrive despite the challenges of kidney disease.

Importance of Nutrition in Managing Kidney Health

Proper nutrition plays a crucial role in managing kidney health, particularly for individuals undergoing dialysis. This section explores the significance of nutrition in supporting kidney function and overall well-being.

1. Nutritional Goals for Kidney Health

Explanation of the specific nutritional goals for individuals with kidney disease, including managing fluid intake, controlling electrolyte levels, and monitoring protein and phosphorus intake.

How achieving these nutritional goals can help slow the progression of kidney disease and minimize complications.

2. Understanding Dietary Restrictions

Overview of common dietary restrictions for individuals undergoing dialysis, such as limitations on sodium, potassium, phosphorus, and fluid intake.

Explanation of how these restrictions help alleviate symptoms and reduce the burden on the kidneys.

3. Balancing Macronutrients

Guidance on achieving a balanced diet that provides adequate protein for muscle maintenance and repair while minimizing the burden on the kidneys.

Tips for balancing carbohydrate and fat intake to support energy levels and overall health.

4. Managing Fluid Intake

Importance of monitoring fluid intake to prevent fluid overload and associated complications such as hypertension, edema, and congestive heart failure.

Strategies for managing thirst and reducing fluid intake without compromising hydration.

5. Minimizing Phosphorus and Potassium

Explanation of the role of phosphorus and potassium in kidney health and why individuals with kidney disease need to limit their intake.

Tips for identifying and avoiding high-phosphorus and high-potassium foods while still enjoying a varied and nutritious diet.

6. Incorporating Kidney-Friendly Foods

Introduction to kidney-friendly foods that are low in sodium, potassium, and phosphorus while still providing essential nutrients.

Suggestions for incorporating fruits, vegetables, whole grains, lean proteins, and healthy fats into your diet.

By understanding the importance of nutrition in managing kidney health and learning how to navigate dietary restrictions, you can take proactive steps to support your overall well-being and improve your quality of life.

How This Book Can Help You

This section highlights the unique features and benefits of this book, explaining how it can serve as an invaluable resource and companion on your kidney dialysis diet journey.

1. Comprehensive Guidance

Overview of the comprehensive information provided in this book, covering everything from the basics of kidney disease and dialysis to practical dietary strategies and delicious recipes.

2. Practical Tips and Advice

Promise of practical tips, advice, and strategies to help you navigate the challenges of managing a kidney-friendly diet in your everyday life.

Suggestions for meal planning, grocery shopping, dining out, and handling social occasions.

3. Delicious and Nutritious Recipes

Description of the wide variety of delicious and nutritious recipes included in this book, designed specifically for individuals undergoing dialysis.

Promise of flavorful meals and snacks that adhere to kidney-friendly dietary guidelines without sacrificing taste or satisfaction.

4. Empowerment and Support

Commitment to empowering you with the knowledge and tools you need to take control of your kidney health and make informed decisions about your diet and lifestyle.

Emphasis on the importance of self-care, advocacy, and building a supportive network of healthcare providers, family, and friends.

Whether you're newly diagnosed with kidney disease or have been managing it for years, this book is designed to be your trusted companion and guide, providing you with the resources and support you need to thrive on your kidney dialysis diet journey.

Chapter 1

Fundamentals of Kidney Health

Kidney dialysis is a life-saving treatment for individuals whose kidneys are no longer able to adequately filter waste products and excess fluid from the blood. This section provides an overview of kidney dialysis, its purpose, types, and considerations for those undergoing this treatment.

1. Purpose of Kidney Dialysis

Explanation of how kidney dialysis functions as an artificial replacement for lost kidney function by removing waste products, excess fluids, and toxins from the bloodstream.

Importance of dialysis in maintaining electrolyte balance, controlling blood pressure, and managing symptoms of kidney failure.

2. Types of Kidney Dialysis

Overview of the two main types of kidney dialysis: hemodialysis and peritoneal dialysis.

Description of hemodialysis, which involves filtering blood through an external machine, and peritoneal dialysis, which uses the lining of the abdomen as a natural filter.

Discussion of the advantages and limitations of each type of dialysis, as well as factors influencing treatment choice.

3. Frequency and Duration of Dialysis

Explanation of the typical schedule for dialysis treatments, including frequency (e.g., three times per week for hemodialysis) and duration (e.g., four to six hours per session for hemodialysis).

Importance of adhering to the prescribed dialysis schedule to maintain stable fluid and electrolyte balance and prevent complications.

4. Preparation and Considerations for Dialysis

Overview of the preparation process for dialysis treatments, including vascular access placement for hemodialysis and training for peritoneal dialysis.

Discussion of lifestyle adjustments and considerations for individuals undergoing dialysis, such as dietary modifications, fluid restrictions, and medication management.

Dietary Goals and Challenges

Maintaining a healthy diet is essential for individuals undergoing kidney dialysis to support treatment effectiveness, manage symptoms, and improve overall well-being. However, there are unique dietary goals and challenges that individuals on dialysis must navigate.

1. Dietary Goals for Dialysis Patients

Explanation of the primary dietary goals for individuals undergoing dialysis, including managing fluid intake, controlling electrolyte levels (e.g., sodium, potassium, phosphorus), and monitoring protein intake.

Importance of achieving these dietary goals to minimize complications, such as fluid overload, electrolyte imbalances, and malnutrition.

2. Challenges of the Dialysis Diet

Discussion of the dietary challenges faced by individuals undergoing dialysis, such as restrictions on high-potassium and high-phosphorus foods, limitations on fluid intake, and the need to monitor protein intake.

Impact of dietary restrictions on food choices, meal planning, and dining out, as well as potential social and emotional challenges associated with dietary modifications.

3. Importance of Nutritional Support

Emphasis on the importance of nutritional support and guidance from healthcare professionals, including registered dietitians specializing in renal nutrition.

Description of the role of dietary education, counseling, and ongoing monitoring in helping individuals on dialysis achieve and maintain optimal nutritional status.

Navigating the dietary goals and challenges of kidney dialysis requires education, support, and careful management. By understanding the purpose of dialysis and the specific dietary goals and challenges associated with treatment, individuals undergoing dialysis can take proactive steps to optimize their nutritional intake and improve their overall health and well-being.

Nutritional Guidelines for Kidney Dialysis Patients

A kidney-friendly diet is designed to help individuals with kidney disease or kidney failure manage their condition effectively by reducing the workload on the kidneys, minimizing the buildup of waste products and excess fluids in the body, and maintaining overall health and well-being. Here's an overview of key principles of a kidney-friendly diet:

1. Moderate Protein Intake: While protein is essential for overall health, excessive protein consumption can burden the kidneys and contribute to waste buildup in the blood. Individuals with kidney disease are typically advised to moderate their protein intake and focus on high-quality protein sources such as lean meats, poultry, fish, eggs, dairy products, and plant-based proteins like beans, lentils, and tofu.

2. Limit Sodium Intake: High sodium intake can lead to fluid retention, high blood pressure, and other complications for individuals with kidney disease. Therefore, it's important to limit the consumption of high-sodium foods such as processed meats, canned soups and vegetables, salty snacks, and fast food. Instead, choose fresh or minimally processed foods and use herbs, spices, and other flavorings to enhance taste without adding extra salt.

3. Control Potassium and Phosphorus: Potassium and phosphorus are electrolytes that can accumulate to dangerous levels in the blood for individuals with kidney disease. To control potassium intake, limit consumption of high-potassium foods such as bananas, oranges, tomatoes, potatoes, and dried fruits. Similarly, restrict phosphorus intake by avoiding processed foods, dairy products, nuts, seeds, and carbonated beverages containing phosphate additives.

4. Monitor Fluid Intake: Individuals with kidney disease may need to restrict their fluid intake to prevent fluid overload and manage symptoms such as swelling, shortness of breath, and high blood pressure. It's important to limit consumption of fluid-rich foods such as soups, ice cream, gelatin desserts, and juicy fruits, and to monitor fluid intake throughout the day.

5. Choose Kidney-Friendly Carbohydrates: Opt for whole grains, fruits, and vegetables as primary sources of carbohydrates in a kidney-friendly diet. These foods provide essential nutrients and fiber while being low in sodium, potassium, and phosphorus. Limit intake of refined carbohydrates and sugary foods and beverages, which can contribute to weight gain and other health problems.

6. Manage Portion Sizes: Pay attention to portion sizes to avoid overeating and prevent excessive calorie intake. Use measuring cups, spoons, or a food scale to measure portions accurately, especially for high-calorie or high-protein foods.

7. Work with a Registered Dietitian: A registered dietitian experienced in renal nutrition can help individuals with kidney disease develop personalized meal plans and dietary strategies tailored to their specific needs and goals. They can provide guidance on food choices, portion control, and meal planning to support kidney health and overall well-being.

Managing Fluid Intake

For individuals with kidney disease, managing fluid intake is essential to prevent fluid overload, maintain electrolyte balance, and manage symptoms such as swelling, high blood pressure, and shortness of breath. Here are some tips for managing fluid intake in a kidney-friendly diet:

1. Set a Fluid Limit: Work with your healthcare provider or dietitian to determine an appropriate fluid intake limit based on your individual needs and health status. This limit may vary depending on factors such as kidney function, urine output, and other medical conditions.

2. Monitor Fluid Intake: Keep track of your fluid intake throughout the day using a diary or mobile app. Be mindful of not only beverages but also fluid-rich foods such as soups, ice cream, gelatin desserts, and juicy fruits.

3. Limit Fluid-Rich Foods: Reduce consumption of foods with high water content, such as soups, stews, sauces, ice cream, gelatin desserts, and juicy fruits like watermelon and oranges. Opt for smaller portions or choose lower-fluid alternatives whenever possible.

4. Choose Thirst-Quenching Alternatives: If you're feeling thirsty between meals, choose thirst-quenching alternatives such as ice chips, sugar-free gum, hard candy, or frozen grapes. These options can help satisfy your thirst without adding extra fluid to your diet.

5. Use Ice Chips: Sucking on ice chips can help relieve thirst and provide oral stimulation without contributing to fluid intake. Keep a supply of ice chips readily available for whenever you need a refreshing treat.

6. Stay Cool: Avoid activities and environments that can lead to excessive sweating and fluid loss. Stay indoors during hot weather, use fans or air conditioning to stay cool, and wear lightweight, breathable clothing to help regulate body temperature.

7. Work with a Dietitian: A registered dietitian can provide personalized guidance on managing fluid intake, including practical tips and strategies for staying within your fluid limit while still meeting your nutritional needs and enjoying a variety of foods and beverages.

By following these strategies and working closely with a healthcare provider or dietitian, individuals with kidney disease can effectively manage fluid intake as part of a kidney-friendly diet, supporting optimal kidney health and overall well-being.

Controlling Sodium Levels

Sodium plays a significant role in fluid balance and blood pressure regulation, but excessive sodium intake can be detrimental to kidney health, especially for individuals with kidney disease. Here's how to control sodium levels in a kidney-friendly diet:

1. Read Food Labels: Check food labels for sodium content and choose products that are lower in sodium. Pay attention to serving sizes and be mindful of hidden sources of sodium in processed and packaged foods.

2. Limit Processed Foods: Processed and packaged foods, such as canned soups, deli meats, frozen dinners, and salty snacks, are often high in sodium. Limit consumption of these foods and choose fresh, whole foods whenever possible.

3. Cook from Scratch: Cooking meals from scratch allows you to control the amount of sodium added to your food. Use fresh or minimally processed ingredients, herbs, spices, and other flavorings to enhance taste without relying on added salt.

4. Choose Low-Sodium Alternatives: Opt for low-sodium or sodium-free versions of condiments, sauces, and seasonings, such as low-sodium soy sauce, broth, and canned vegetables. Look for products labeled "no added salt" or "sodium-free" when shopping.

5. Rinse Canned Foods: If using canned foods, such as beans, vegetables, or tuna, rinse them under cold water before use to remove excess sodium from the surface.

6. Be Careful with Condiments: Condiments like ketchup, mustard, barbecue sauce, and salad dressings can be sources of hidden sodium. Choose low-sodium or homemade versions, or use them sparingly to control sodium intake.

7. Limit Restaurant Meals: Restaurant meals are often high in sodium, as chefs use salt to enhance flavor. Limit dining out or choose restaurants that offer lower-sodium options, and ask for sauces and dressings on the side so you can control how much you use.

8. Gradually Reduce Salt: Gradually reduce the amount of salt you add to your meals to allow your taste buds to adjust to lower sodium levels. Experiment with herbs, spices, lemon juice, vinegar, and other flavorings to enhance taste without relying on salt.

By following these tips and making smart food choices, individuals with kidney disease can effectively control sodium levels in their diet, support kidney health, and reduce the risk of complications such as fluid retention, high blood pressure, and

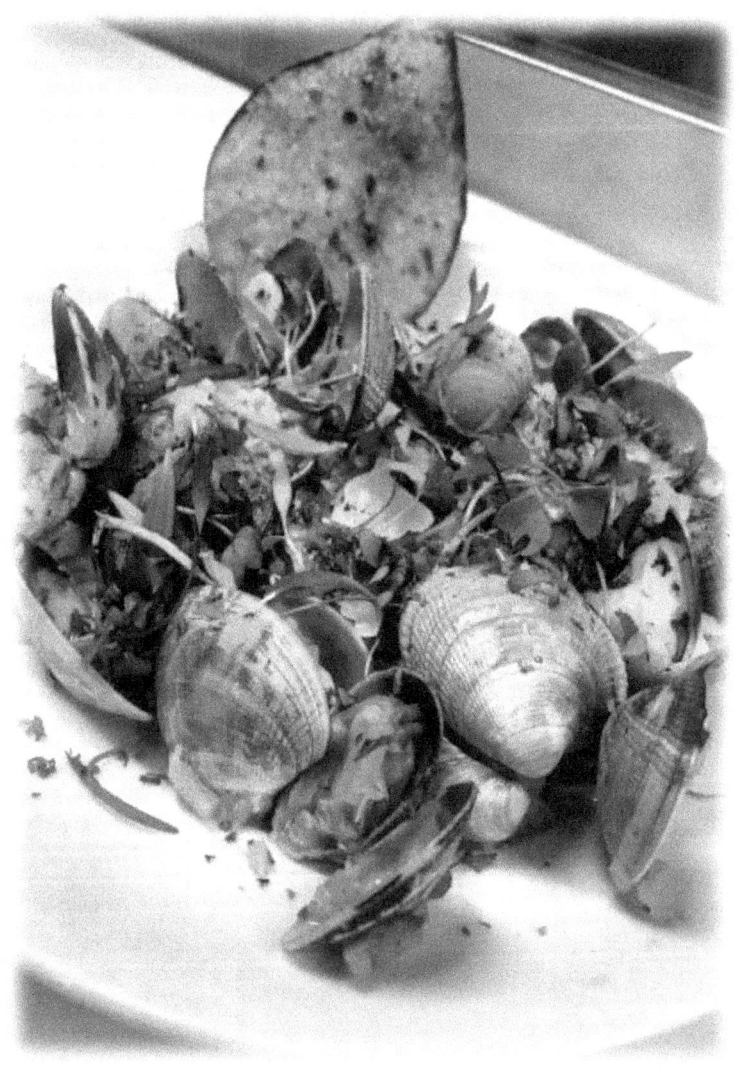

Chapter 2

30-Day Meal Plan for a Kidney Dialysis Diet

This plan focuses on incorporating foods rich in healthy fats, fiber, low sodium and low potassium while limiting saturated fats, trans fats, and refined carbohydrates. It also includes a variety of fruits, vegetables, whole grains, and low-fat dairy products to promote overall health of your kidney.

Day 1:

- Breakfast: Scrambled eggs with spinach, whole grain toast, and sliced strawberries.

- Lunch: Grilled chicken salad with mixed greens, cherry tomatoes, cucumbers, and a vinaigrette dressing.

- Snack: Greek yogurt with a sprinkle of crushed nuts.

- Dinner: Baked salmon, quinoa, steamed broccoli, and a side of roasted sweet potatoes.

Day 2:

- Breakfast: Oatmeal with sliced banana and a drizzle of honey.

- Lunch: Lentil soup with a side of whole grain crackers.

- Snack: Fresh apple slices with a small portion of cheese.

- Dinner: Turkey meatballs, whole wheat pasta, tomato sauce, and a side of sautéed zucchini.

Day 3:

- Breakfast: Smoothie with berries, low-fat yogurt, and a splash of almond milk.

- Lunch: Tuna salad with mixed greens, cherry tomatoes, and whole grain bread.

- Snack: Carrot and cucumber sticks with hummus.

- Dinner: Grilled shrimp, quinoa, asparagus, and a side of mixed berries.

Day 4:

- Breakfast: Whole grain bagel with cream cheese and sliced strawberries.

- Lunch: Chicken and vegetable stir-fry with brown rice.

- Snack: Cottage cheese with pineapple chunks.

- Dinner: Baked cod, roasted sweet potatoes, green beans, and a side of watermelon.

Day 5:

- Breakfast: Greek yogurt parfait with granola and mixed berries.

- Lunch: Spinach and feta stuffed chicken breast, quinoa, and steamed broccoli.

- Snack: Handful of mixed nuts.

- Dinner: Beef and vegetable kebabs, brown rice, and a side salad with vinaigrette.

Day 6:

- Breakfast: Whole grain toast with avocado and poached eggs.

- Lunch: Minestrone soup with a side of whole grain bread.

- Snack: Sliced pear with a small portion of low-fat cheese.

- Dinner: Grilled tilapia, wild rice, sautéed spinach, and a side of melon.

Day 7:

- Breakfast: Cottage cheese pancakes with fresh berries.

- Lunch: Turkey and vegetable wrap with a side of sliced cucumber.

- Snack: Orange slices with a handful of almonds.

- Dinner: Stir-fried tofu with mixed vegetables, quinoa, and a side of sliced strawberries.

Day 8:

- Breakfast: Veggie omelet with bell peppers, onions, and tomatoes, served with whole grain toast.

- Lunch: Quinoa salad with black beans, corn, cherry tomatoes, and a lime-cilantro dressing.

- Snack: Celery sticks with peanut butter.

- Dinner: Grilled chicken breast, roasted Brussels sprouts, and mashed sweet potatoes.

Day 9:

- Breakfast: Overnight oats made with almond milk, topped with sliced peaches and a sprinkle of cinnamon.

- Lunch: Spinach and strawberry salad with grilled chicken and balsamic vinaigrette.

- Snack: Sliced cucumbers with tzatziki sauce.

- Dinner: Baked cod with lemon and herbs, quinoa pilaf, and steamed asparagus.

Day 10:

- Breakfast: Greek yogurt with honey, granola, and mixed berries.

- Lunch: Turkey and avocado wrap with whole grain tortilla and a side of carrot sticks.

- Snack: Handful of trail mix (unsalted nuts and dried fruits).

- Dinner: Beef and vegetable stir-fry with brown rice.

Day 11:

- Breakfast: Whole grain waffle topped with almond butter and sliced bananas.

- Lunch: Lentil and vegetable soup with a side of whole grain crackers.

- Snack: Cherry tomatoes with mozzarella cheese balls.

- Dinner: Grilled salmon, quinoa, roasted cauliflower, and a side of watermelon cubes.

Day 12:

- Breakfast: Scrambled tofu with sautéed spinach and whole grain toast.

- Lunch: Chickpea and vegetable salad with lemon-tahini dressing.

- Snack: Apple slices with a small portion of cheese.

- Dinner: Turkey meatloaf, roasted sweet potatoes, green beans, and a side of sliced strawberries.

Day 13:

- Breakfast: Smoothie bowl made with mixed berries, spinach, almond milk, and a sprinkle of chia seeds.

- Lunch: Chicken Caesar salad with grilled chicken breast, romaine lettuce, and homemade Caesar dressing.

- Snack: Carrot and celery sticks with hummus.

- Dinner: Grilled shrimp skewers, quinoa, sautéed kale, and a side of melon slices.

Day 14:

- Breakfast: Whole grain English muffin with scrambled eggs and avocado slices.

- Lunch: Caprese salad with fresh mozzarella, tomato slices, basil leaves, and balsamic glaze.

- Snack: Greek yogurt with sliced peaches.

- Dinner: Baked chicken thighs, brown rice pilaf, roasted broccoli, and a side of mixed berries.

Day 15:

- Breakfast: Banana almond smoothie made with almond milk, Greek yogurt, and a scoop of almond butter.

- Lunch: Turkey and vegetable stir-fry with brown rice.

- Snack: Handful of mixed nuts.

- Dinner: Baked cod with lemon and herbs, quinoa, steamed asparagus, and a side of pineapple chunks.

Day 16:

- Breakfast: Whole grain toast with avocado mash and poached eggs.

- Lunch: Lentil and vegetable soup with a side of whole grain crackers.

- Snack: Sliced cucumber with hummus.

- Dinner: Grilled salmon, quinoa pilaf, roasted Brussels sprouts, and a side of mixed berries.

Day 17:

- Breakfast: Greek yogurt parfait with granola and mixed berries.

- Lunch: Spinach and feta stuffed chicken breast, quinoa, steamed broccoli, and a side of sliced watermelon.

- Snack: Apple slices with a small portion of cheese.

- Dinner: Beef and vegetable kebabs, brown rice, and a side salad with balsamic vinaigrette.

Day 18:

- Breakfast: Whole grain bagel with cream cheese and sliced strawberries.

- Lunch: Chicken and vegetable stir-fry with brown rice.

- Snack: Carrot and celery sticks with hummus.

- Dinner: Grilled tilapia, wild rice pilaf, sautéed spinach, and a side of cantaloupe slices.

Day 19:

- Breakfast: Cottage cheese pancakes with fresh berries.

- Lunch: Turkey and avocado wrap with whole grain tortilla and a side of carrot sticks.

- Snack: Handful of trail mix (unsalted nuts and dried fruits).

- Dinner: Baked chicken thighs, quinoa, roasted cauliflower, and a side of mixed berries.

Day 20:

- Breakfast: Smoothie bowl made with mixed berries, spinach, almond milk, and a sprinkle of chia seeds.

- Lunch: Chickpea and vegetable salad with lemon-tahini dressing.

- Snack: Sliced cucumber with tzatziki sauce.

- Dinner: Grilled shrimp skewers, quinoa, sautéed kale, and a side of peach slices.

Day 21:

- Breakfast: Scrambled tofu with sautéed spinach and whole grain toast.

- Lunch: Greek salad with mixed greens, cucumbers, tomatoes, olives, feta cheese, and a lemon-herb dressing.

- Snack: Handful of almonds.

- Dinner: Baked cod with lemon and herbs, brown rice, steamed asparagus, and a side of mixed berries.

Day 22:

- Breakfast: Whole grain waffle topped with almond butter and sliced bananas.

- Lunch: Lentil and vegetable soup with a side of whole grain crackers.

- Snack: Greek yogurt with honey and mixed berries.

- Dinner: Turkey meatloaf, roasted sweet potatoes, green beans, and a side of pineapple chunks.

Day 23:

- Breakfast: Overnight oats made with almond milk, topped with sliced peaches and a sprinkle of cinnamon.

- Lunch: Spinach and strawberry salad with grilled chicken breast and balsamic vinaigrette.

- Snack: Celery sticks with peanut butter.

- Dinner: Grilled salmon, quinoa pilaf, roasted Brussels sprouts, and a side of sliced strawberries.

Day 24:

- Breakfast: Smoothie with berries, low-fat yogurt, and a splash of almond milk.

- Lunch: Turkey and vegetable stir-fry with brown rice.

- Snack: Cottage cheese with pineapple chunks.

- Dinner: Beef and vegetable kebabs, brown rice, and a side salad with vinaigrette dressing.

Day 25:

- Breakfast: Whole grain toast with avocado mash and poached eggs.

- Lunch: Lentil and vegetable soup with a side of whole grain crackers.

- Snack: Sliced cucumber with hummus.

- Dinner: Grilled salmon, quinoa pilaf, roasted Brussels sprouts, and a side of mixed berries.

Day 26:

- Breakfast: Greek yogurt parfait with granola and mixed berries.

- Lunch: Spinach and feta stuffed chicken breast, quinoa, steamed broccoli, and a side of sliced watermelon.

- Snack: Apple slices with a small portion of cheese.

- Dinner: Beef and vegetable kebabs, brown rice, and a side salad with balsamic vinaigrette.

Day 27:

- Breakfast: Whole grain bagel with cream cheese and sliced strawberries.

- Lunch: Chicken and vegetable stir-fry with brown rice.

- Snack: Carrot and celery sticks with hummus.

- Dinner: Grilled tilapia, wild rice pilaf, sautéed spinach, and a side of cantaloupe slices.

Day 28:

- Breakfast: Cottage cheese pancakes with fresh berries.

- Lunch: Turkey and avocado wrap with whole grain tortilla and a side of carrot sticks.

- Snack: Handful of trail mix (unsalted nuts and dried fruits).

- Dinner: Baked chicken thighs, quinoa, roasted cauliflower, and a side of mixed berries.

Day 29:

- Breakfast: Smoothie bowl made with mixed berries, spinach, almond milk, and a sprinkle of chia seeds.

- Lunch: Chickpea and vegetable salad with lemon-tahini dressing.

- Snack: Sliced cucumber with tzatziki sauce.

- Dinner: Grilled shrimp skewers, quinoa, sautéed kale, and a side of peach slices.

Day 30:

- Breakfast: Scrambled tofu with sautéed spinach and whole grain toast.

- Lunch: Greek salad with mixed greens, cucumbers, tomatoes, olives, feta cheese, and a lemon-herb dressing.

- Snack: Handful of almonds.

- Dinner: Baked cod with lemon and herbs, brown rice, steamed asparagus, and a side of mixed berries.

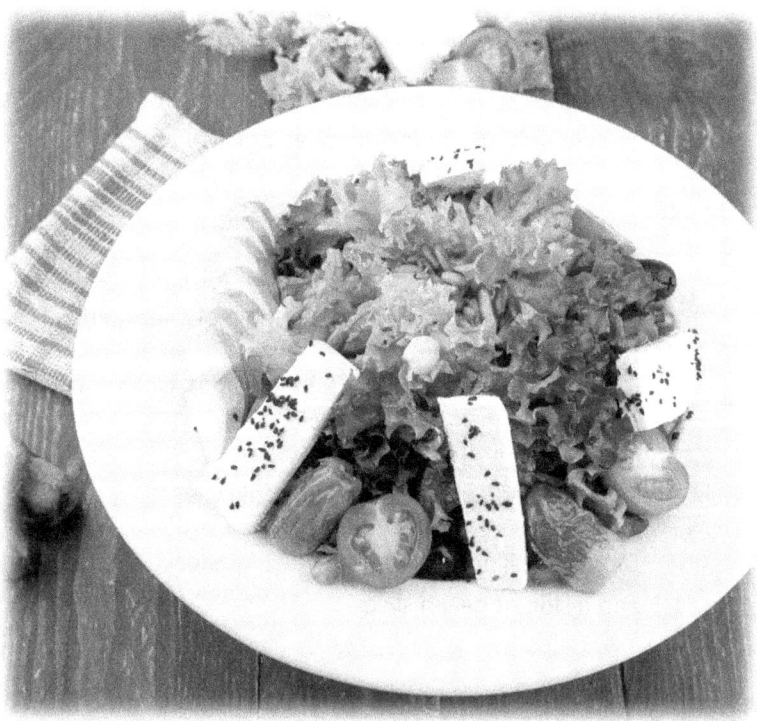

Chapter 3

Nutritious and Delicious Breakfast Options to Start your Day Right

These kidney-friendly breakfast recipes are not only delicious but also provide essential nutrients while adhering to dietary restrictions for individuals undergoing kidney dialysis. Adjust ingredients and portion sizes as needed to suit individual dietary requirements and preferences.

1. Vegetable and Cheese Omelet

Ingredients:

- 2 large eggs

- 1/4 cup chopped bell peppers

- 1/4 cup chopped onions

- 1/4 cup chopped tomatoes

- 2 tablespoons shredded low-fat cheese

- Salt and pepper to taste

- Cooking spray or olive oil for greasing

Preparation:

1. In a bowl, beat the eggs until well combined. Season with salt and pepper.

2. Heat a non-stick skillet over medium heat and coat with cooking spray or olive oil.

3. Add the bell peppers and onions to the skillet and cook until softened, about 2-3 minutes.

4. Pour the beaten eggs into the skillet, swirling to evenly distribute the vegetables.

5. Allow the eggs to cook undisturbed until the edges begin to set, then gently lift the edges with a spatula to let the uncooked eggs flow underneath.

6. Sprinkle the chopped tomatoes and shredded cheese over one half of the omelet.

7. Carefully fold the other half of the omelet over the filling and cook for an additional 1-2 minutes, or until the cheese is melted and the eggs are cooked through.

8. Slide the omelet onto a plate and serve hot.

2. Berry and Yogurt Parfait

Ingredients:

- 1/2 cup plain Greek yogurt

- 1/4 cup low-sugar granola

- 1/4 cup mixed berries (such as strawberries, blueberries, and raspberries)

- 1 tablespoon honey (optional)

Preparation:

1. In a serving glass or bowl, layer the Greek yogurt, granola, and mixed berries.

2. Drizzle with honey, if desired, for added sweetness.

3. Repeat the layers until all ingredients are used, ending with a layer of berries on top.

4. Serve immediately as a nutritious and satisfying breakfast option.

3. Spinach and Mushroom Scramble

Ingredients:

- 2 large eggs

- 1/4 cup chopped spinach

- 1/4 cup sliced mushrooms

- 1 tablespoon chopped onions

- Salt and pepper to taste

- Cooking spray or olive oil for greasing

Preparation:

1. In a bowl, beat the eggs until well combined. Season with salt and pepper.

2. Heat a non-stick skillet over medium heat and coat with cooking spray or olive oil.

3. Add the chopped onions and sliced mushrooms to the skillet and cook until softened, about 2-3 minutes.

4. Add the chopped spinach to the skillet and cook until wilted, about 1-2 minutes.

5. Pour the beaten eggs into the skillet, swirling to evenly distribute the vegetables.

6. Allow the eggs to cook undisturbed until the edges begin to set, then gently scramble with a spatula until cooked through.

7. Transfer the scramble to a plate and serve hot.

4. Overnight Oats with Mixed Berries

Ingredients:

- 1/2 cup rolled oats

- 1/2 cup almond milk (or any milk of your choice)

- 1/4 cup plain Greek yogurt

- 1/4 cup mixed berries (such as strawberries, blueberries, and raspberries)

- 1 tablespoon chia seeds (optional)

- 1 tablespoon honey (optional)

Preparation:

1. In a mason jar or bowl, combine the rolled oats, almond milk, Greek yogurt, mixed berries, and chia seeds.

2. Stir well to combine all ingredients.

3. Cover the jar or bowl and refrigerate overnight, or for at least 4 hours, to allow the oats to soak and soften.

4. Before serving, stir the mixture again and add honey, if desired, for added sweetness.

5. Enjoy cold or at room temperature as a convenient and nutritious breakfast option.

5. Whole Grain Toast with Avocado Mash and Poached Egg

Ingredients:

- 1 slice whole grain bread, toasted
- 1/2 ripe avocado
- 1 large egg
- Salt and pepper to taste

Preparation:

1. Mash the ripe avocado in a small bowl with a fork until smooth. Season with salt and pepper to taste.

2. Poach the egg by bringing a pot of water to a gentle simmer. Crack the egg into a small bowl and carefully slide it into the simmering water. Cook for 3-4 minutes, or until the egg white is set but the yolk is still runny.

3. While the egg is poaching, toast the whole grain bread until golden brown.

4. Spread the mashed avocado evenly onto the toasted bread.

5. Using a slotted spoon, carefully remove the poached egg from the water and place it on top of the avocado mash.

6. Season the poached egg with additional salt and pepper, if desired.

7. Serve immediately as a delicious and nutrient-rich breakfast option.

6. Fruit and Nut Breakfast Bowl

Ingredients:

- 1/2 cup cooked quinoa

- 1/4 cup sliced almonds

- 1/4 cup diced apples

- 1/4 cup diced peaches

- 1 tablespoon honey (optional)

- 1/4 teaspoon cinnamon

Preparation:

1. In a bowl, combine the cooked quinoa, sliced almonds, diced apples, and diced peaches.

2. Drizzle honey over the mixture, if desired, and sprinkle with cinnamon.

3. Stir well to combine all ingredients.

4. Serve immediately as a hearty and nutritious breakfast bowl.

7. Cottage Cheese Pancakes

Ingredients:

- 1/2 cup cottage cheese

- 2 large eggs

- 1/4 cup whole wheat flour

- 1/4 teaspoon baking powder

- 1/4 teaspoon vanilla extract

- Cooking spray or olive oil for greasing

Preparation:

1. In a blender or food processor, combine the cottage cheese, eggs, whole wheat flour, baking powder, and vanilla extract. Blend until smooth.

2. Heat a non-stick skillet over medium heat and coat with cooking spray or olive oil.

3. Pour small portions of the pancake batter onto the skillet to form pancakes.

4. Cook for 2-3 minutes on each side, or until golden brown and cooked through.

5. Serve hot with your choice of toppings, such as fresh fruit or a drizzle of honey.

8. Breakfast Burrito

Ingredients:

- 1 whole grain tortilla

- 2 large eggs, scrambled

- 1/4 cup black beans, drained and rinsed

- 1/4 cup diced tomatoes

- 2 tablespoons shredded low-fat cheese

- Salsa and avocado slices for topping

Preparation:

1. Warm the whole grain tortilla in a skillet or microwave until soft and pliable.

2. Fill the tortilla with scrambled eggs, black beans, diced tomatoes, and shredded cheese.

3. Roll up the tortilla to form a burrito.

4. Serve topped with salsa and avocado slices for added flavor and nutrition.

9. Spinach and Mushroom Frittata

Ingredients:

- 4 large eggs

- 1/4 cup chopped spinach

- 1/4 cup sliced mushrooms

- 2 tablespoons chopped onions

- 2 tablespoons shredded low-fat cheese

- Salt and pepper to taste

- Cooking spray or olive oil for greasing

Preparation:

1. Preheat the oven to 350°F (175°C).

2. In a bowl, beat the eggs until well combined. Season with salt and pepper.

3. Heat a non-stick skillet over medium heat and coat with cooking spray or olive oil.

4. Add the chopped onions and sliced mushrooms to the skillet and cook until softened, about 2-3 minutes.

5. Add the chopped spinach to the skillet and cook until wilted, about 1-2 minutes.

6. Pour the beaten eggs into the skillet, swirling to evenly distribute the vegetables.

7. Sprinkle the shredded cheese over the top of the frittata.

8. Transfer the skillet to the preheated oven and bake for 10-12 minutes, or until the eggs are set and the cheese is melted.

9. Slice into wedges and serve hot.

10. Banana Almond Smoothie

Ingredients:

- 1 ripe banana
- 1 cup almond milk (or any milk of your choice)
- 2 tablespoons almond butter
- 1 tablespoon honey (optional)
- 1/4 teaspoon cinnamon
- Ice cubes (optional)

Preparation:

1. In a blender, combine the ripe banana, almond milk, almond butter, honey (if using), and cinnamon.

2. Add ice cubes, if desired, to make the smoothie colder and thicker.

3. Blend until smooth and creamy.

4. Pour into a glass and serve immediately as a refreshing and nutrient-rich breakfast smoothie.

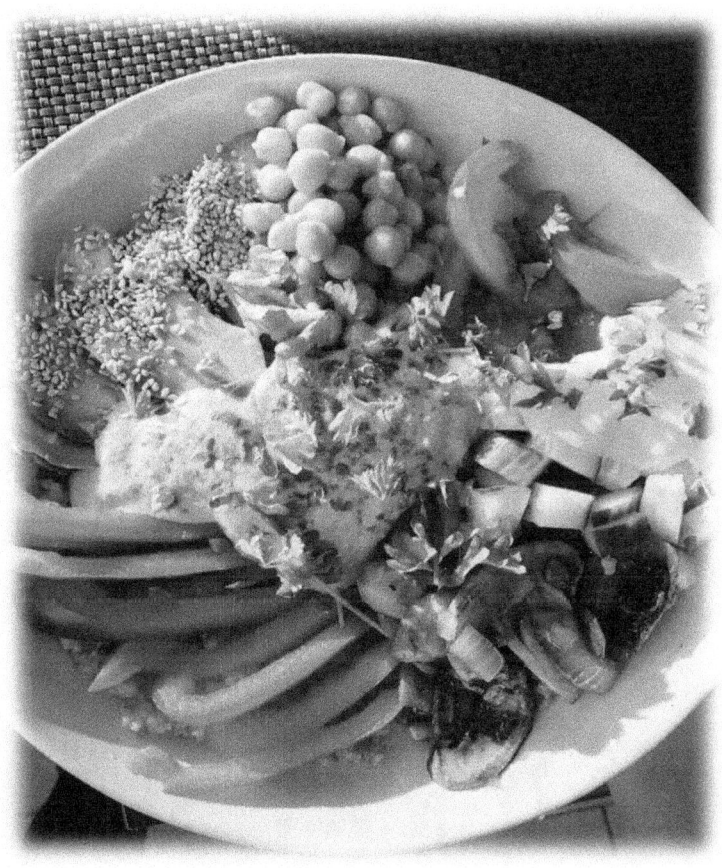

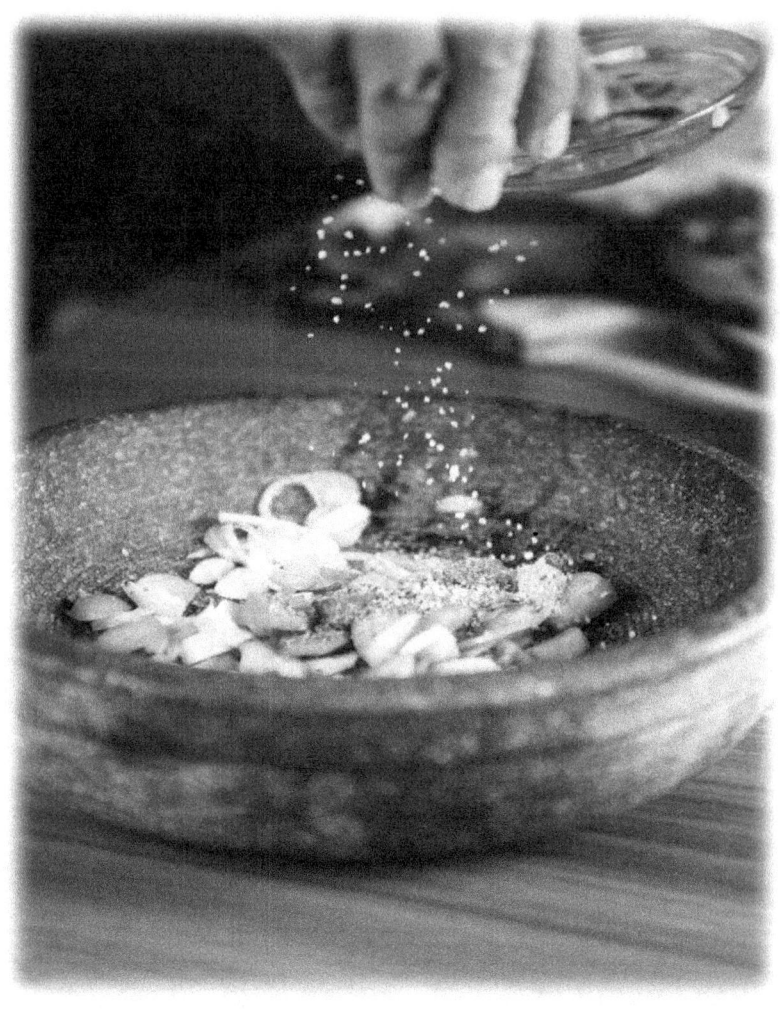

Chapter 4

Quick and Healthy Lunch Ideas for Busy Days

These satisfying lunch recipes are not only delicious but also kidney-friendly, providing essential nutrients while adhering to dietary restrictions for individuals undergoing kidney dialysis. Adjust ingredients and portion sizes as needed to suit individual dietary requirements and preferences. Enjoy these flavorful and nutritious lunch options as part of a balanced diet.

1. Grilled Chicken Salad

Ingredients:

- 4 oz grilled chicken breast, sliced

- 2 cups mixed salad greens (such as spinach, arugula, and romaine lettuce)

- 1/4 cup cherry tomatoes, halved

- 1/4 cup cucumber, sliced

- 1/4 cup bell peppers, diced

- 2 tablespoons balsamic vinaigrette dressing

Preparation:

1. Season the chicken breast with salt and pepper, then grill until cooked through. Let it rest for a few minutes before slicing.

2. In a large bowl, combine the mixed salad greens, cherry tomatoes, cucumber, and bell peppers.

3. Add the sliced grilled chicken on top of the salad.

4. Drizzle with balsamic vinaigrette dressing and toss gently to coat.

5. Serve immediately as a satisfying and nutritious lunch option.

2. Lentil and Vegetable Soup

Ingredients:

- 1 cup dried lentils, rinsed and drained

- 4 cups low-sodium vegetable broth

- 1 onion, diced

- 2 carrots, diced

- 2 celery stalks, diced

- 2 garlic cloves, minced

- 1 teaspoon dried thyme

- Salt and pepper to taste

- Fresh parsley for garnish (optional)

Preparation:

1. In a large pot, combine the dried lentils, vegetable broth, diced onion, carrots, celery, minced garlic, and dried thyme.

2. Bring the mixture to a boil, then reduce the heat to low and simmer for about 20-25 minutes, or until the lentils and vegetables are tender.

3. Season with salt and pepper to taste.

4. Ladle the soup into bowls and garnish with fresh parsley, if desired.

5. Serve hot with a slice of whole grain bread for a hearty and satisfying lunch.

3. Turkey and Avocado Wrap

Ingredients:

- 1 whole grain tortilla

- 3 oz deli turkey breast slices

- 1/4 avocado, sliced

- 1/4 cup mixed salad greens

- 1 tablespoon hummus

- 1 tablespoon Greek yogurt

- Salt and pepper to taste

Preparation:

1. Lay the whole grain tortilla flat on a clean surface.

2. Spread the hummus evenly over the tortilla, leaving a border around the edges.

3. Layer the deli turkey breast slices, sliced avocado, and mixed salad greens on top of the hummus.

4. Drizzle with Greek yogurt and season with salt and pepper to taste.

5. Roll up the tortilla tightly to form a wrap.

6. Slice the wrap in half diagonally and serve immediately as a delicious and satisfying lunch option.

4. Quinoa and Black Bean Salad

Ingredients:

- 1 cup cooked quinoa

- 1/2 cup canned black beans, drained and rinsed

- 1/4 cup corn kernels (fresh, frozen, or canned)

- 1/4 cup diced tomatoes

- 2 tablespoons chopped red onion

- 2 tablespoons chopped cilantro

- Juice of 1 lime

- Salt and pepper to taste

Preparation:

1. In a large bowl, combine the cooked quinoa, black beans, corn kernels, diced tomatoes, chopped red onion, and chopped cilantro.

2. Squeeze the lime juice over the salad and toss gently to combine.

3. Season with salt and pepper to taste.

4. Serve chilled or at room temperature as a nutritious and satisfying lunch option.

5. Tuna and White Bean Salad

Ingredients:

- 1 can (5 oz) tuna in water, drained

- 1/2 cup canned white beans, drained and rinsed

- 1/4 cup diced cucumber

- 1/4 cup diced bell peppers (any color)

- 2 tablespoons chopped red onion

- 2 tablespoons chopped parsley

- 1 tablespoon olive oil

- 1 tablespoon lemon juice

- Salt and pepper to taste

Preparation:

1. In a large bowl, combine the drained tuna, white beans, diced cucumber, diced bell peppers, chopped red onion, and chopped parsley.

2. Drizzle with olive oil and lemon juice, then toss gently to combine.

3. Season with salt and pepper to taste.

4. Serve chilled or at room temperature as a protein-packed and satisfying lunch option.

6. Baked Salmon with Quinoa and Steamed Vegetables

Ingredients:

- 4 oz salmon fillet
- 1/2 cup cooked quinoa
- 1 cup mixed vegetables (such as broccoli, carrots, and bell peppers)
- 1 tablespoon olive oil
- Salt and pepper to taste
- Lemon wedges for serving

Preparation:

1. Preheat the oven to 400°F (200°C).

2. Place the salmon fillet on a baking sheet lined with parchment paper. Drizzle with olive oil and season with salt and pepper.

3. Bake in the preheated oven for 12-15 minutes, or until the salmon is cooked through and flakes easily with a fork.

4. Meanwhile, steam the mixed vegetables until tender.

5. Serve the baked salmon with cooked quinoa and steamed vegetables. Squeeze fresh lemon juice over the salmon before serving.

7. Veggie and Hummus Wrap

Ingredients:

- 1 whole grain tortilla

- 2 tablespoons hummus

- 1/4 cup shredded carrots

- 1/4 cup sliced cucumber

- 1/4 cup mixed salad greens

- 2 tablespoons crumbled feta cheese

- Salt and pepper to taste

Preparation:

1. Spread the hummus evenly over the whole grain tortilla.

2. Layer the shredded carrots, sliced cucumber, mixed salad greens, and crumbled feta cheese on top of the hummus.

3. Season with salt and pepper to taste.

4. Roll up the tortilla tightly to form a wrap.

5. Slice the wrap in half diagonally and serve immediately.

8. Egg Salad Lettuce Wraps

Ingredients:

- 2 hard-boiled eggs, chopped
- 2 tablespoons Greek yogurt
- 1 tablespoon Dijon mustard
- 1 tablespoon chopped chives
- Salt and pepper to taste
- 4 large lettuce leaves (such as romaine or butter lettuce)
- Sliced tomatoes and avocado for serving

Preparation:

1. In a bowl, combine the chopped hard-boiled eggs, Greek yogurt, Dijon mustard, chopped chives, salt, and pepper.

2. Mix until well combined.

3. Place a spoonful of the egg salad mixture onto each lettuce leaf.

4. Top with sliced tomatoes and avocado.

5. Roll up the lettuce leaves to form wraps and serve immediately.

9. Quinoa and Vegetable Stir-Fry

Ingredients:

- 1/2 cup cooked quinoa

- 1 cup mixed vegetables (such as bell peppers, broccoli, snap peas, and carrots)

- 2 tablespoons low-sodium soy sauce

- 1 tablespoon sesame oil

- 1 clove garlic, minced

- 1 teaspoon grated ginger

- Sesame seeds for garnish (optional)

Preparation:

1. Heat sesame oil in a large skillet or wok over medium-high heat.

2. Add minced garlic and grated ginger to the skillet and cook until fragrant.

3. Add the mixed vegetables to the skillet and stir-fry until tender-crisp.

4. Stir in cooked quinoa and low-sodium soy sauce. Cook for an additional 2-3 minutes, stirring frequently.

5. Remove from heat and garnish with sesame seeds, if desired. Serve hot.

10. Turkey and Veggie Wrap

Ingredients:

- 1 whole grain tortilla

- 3 oz deli turkey breast slices

- 1/4 cup shredded lettuce

- 1/4 cup diced tomatoes

- 1/4 cup diced cucumbers

- 2 tablespoons mashed avocado

- Salt and pepper to taste

Preparation:

1. Lay the whole grain tortilla flat on a clean surface.

2. Layer the deli turkey breast slices, shredded lettuce, diced tomatoes, and diced cucumbers on top of the tortilla.

3. Spread mashed avocado evenly over the ingredients.

4. Season with salt and pepper to taste.

5. Roll up the tortilla tightly to form a wrap.

6. Slice the wrap in half diagonally and serve immediately.

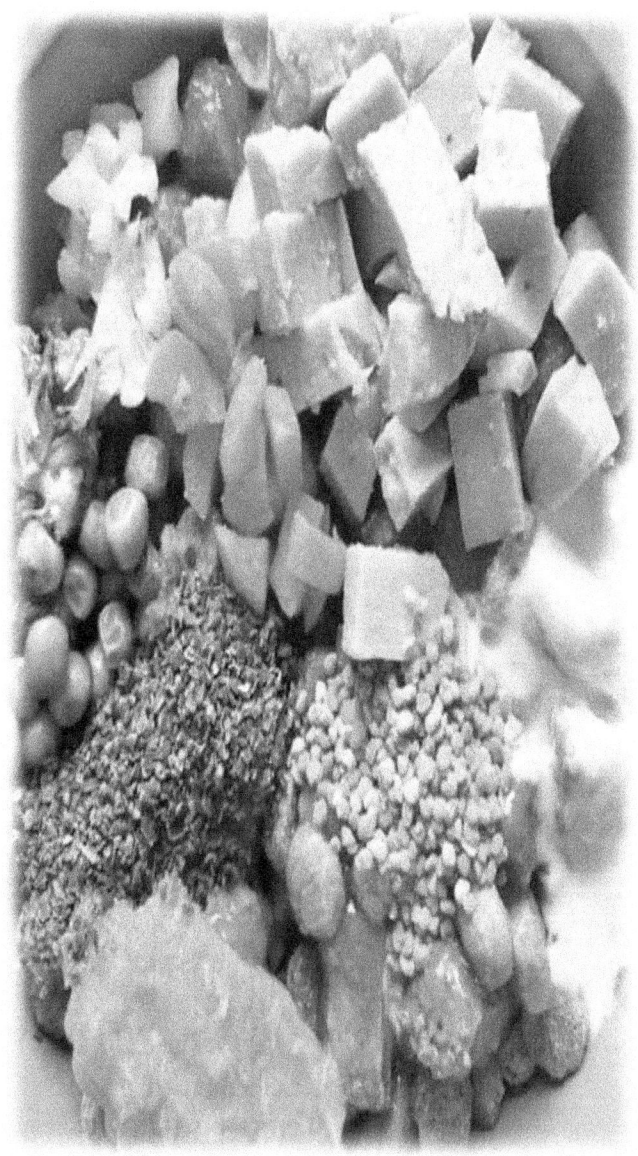

Chapter 5

Nourishing Dinners for Healthy Aging

These dinner ideas provide a variety of flavors and textures, making them suitable for a Kidney Dialysis diet. Feel free to adapt these recipes based on your preferences and dietary needs.

1. Baked Herb-Crusted Chicken with Roasted Vegetables

Ingredients:

- 4 boneless, skinless chicken breasts

- 2 tablespoons olive oil

- 1 tablespoon fresh chopped herbs (such as rosemary, thyme, and parsley)

- 1 teaspoon garlic powder

- Salt and pepper to taste

- 2 cups mixed vegetables (such as carrots, bell peppers, and zucchini), chopped

Preparation:

1. Preheat the oven to 400°F (200°C).

2. In a small bowl, mix together olive oil, chopped herbs, garlic powder, salt, and pepper.

3. Place the chicken breasts on a baking sheet lined with parchment paper.

4. Brush the herb mixture over the chicken breasts, coating them evenly.

5. Arrange the chopped vegetables around the chicken on the baking sheet.

6. Bake in the preheated oven for 20-25 minutes, or until the chicken is cooked through and the vegetables are tender.

7. Serve hot, garnished with additional fresh herbs if desired.

2. Grilled Salmon with Lemon-Dill Sauce and Quinoa Pilaf

Ingredients:

- 4 salmon fillets

- 2 tablespoons olive oil

- 1 tablespoon fresh lemon juice

- 1 teaspoon dried dill

- Salt and pepper to taste

- 1 cup quinoa, rinsed

- 2 cups low-sodium chicken or vegetable broth

- 1 tablespoon chopped fresh parsley (for garnish)

Preparation:

1. Preheat the grill to medium-high heat.

2. In a small bowl, whisk together olive oil, lemon juice, dried dill, salt, and pepper.

3. Brush the salmon fillets with the lemon-dill mixture, coating them evenly.

4. Grill the salmon fillets for 4-5 minutes per side, or until cooked through and flaky.

5. Meanwhile, in a saucepan, bring the chicken or vegetable broth to a boil.

6. Add the rinsed quinoa to the boiling broth, reduce the heat to low, cover, and simmer for 15-20 minutes, or until the quinoa is cooked and the liquid is absorbed.

7. Serve the grilled salmon with quinoa pilaf, garnished with chopped fresh parsley.

3. Vegetarian Stuffed Bell Peppers

Ingredients:

- 4 large bell peppers, halved and seeds removed

- 1 cup cooked brown rice

- 1 can (15 oz) black beans, drained and rinsed

- 1 cup corn kernels (fresh, frozen, or canned)

- 1 cup diced tomatoes

- 1/2 cup shredded cheese (such as cheddar or mozzarella)

- 1 teaspoon chili powder

- 1/2 teaspoon cumin

- Salt and pepper to taste

Preparation:

1. Preheat the oven to 375°F (190°C).

2. In a large bowl, combine cooked brown rice, black beans, corn kernels, diced tomatoes, shredded cheese, chili powder, cumin, salt, and pepper.

3. Fill each bell pepper half with the rice and bean mixture, pressing down gently to pack it in.

4. Place the stuffed bell peppers in a baking dish, cut side up.

5. Cover the dish with aluminum foil and bake in the preheated oven for 30 minutes.

6. Remove the foil and bake for an additional 10-15 minutes, or until the peppers are tender and the filling is heated through.

7. Serve hot, garnished with additional shredded cheese if desired.

4. Lemon Garlic Shrimp Pasta

Ingredients:

- 8 oz whole wheat spaghetti

- 1 lb large shrimp, peeled and deveined

- 2 tablespoons olive oil

- 3 cloves garlic, minced

- Zest and juice of 1 lemon

- 1/4 cup chopped fresh parsley

- Salt and pepper to taste

- Grated Parmesan cheese for serving (optional)

Preparation:

1. Cook the whole wheat spaghetti according to the package instructions until al dente. Drain and set aside.

2. In a large skillet, heat olive oil over medium heat. Add minced garlic and cook until fragrant, about 1-2 minutes.

3. Add the shrimp to the skillet and cook until pink and opaque, about 2-3 minutes per side.

4. Stir in the lemon zest, lemon juice, chopped parsley, cooked spaghetti, salt, and pepper. Toss until everything is well combined and heated through.

5. Serve hot, garnished with grated Parmesan cheese if desired.

5. Baked Cod with Tomato and Herb Salsa

Ingredients:

- 4 cod fillets

- 2 tablespoons olive oil

- 2 cups cherry tomatoes, halved

- 2 cloves garlic, minced

- 1/4 cup chopped fresh basil

- 1/4 cup chopped fresh parsley

- Salt and pepper to taste

- Lemon wedges for serving

Preparation:

1. Preheat the oven to 400°F (200°C).

2. Place the cod fillets on a baking sheet lined with parchment paper. Drizzle with olive oil and season with salt and pepper.

3. In a bowl, toss together cherry tomatoes, minced garlic, chopped basil, chopped parsley, salt, and pepper.

4. Spoon the tomato and herb mixture over the cod fillets.

5. Bake in the preheated oven for 15-20 minutes, or until the cod is cooked through and flakes easily with a fork.

6. Serve hot, with lemon wedges for squeezing over the fish.

6. Vegetable Stir-Fry with Tofu

Ingredients:

- 1 block (14 oz) firm tofu, drained and cubed

- 2 tablespoons soy sauce

- 1 tablespoon sesame oil

- 1 tablespoon cornstarch

- 1 tablespoon vegetable oil

- 2 cups mixed vegetables (such as bell peppers, broccoli, snap peas, and carrots)

- 2 cloves garlic, minced

- 1 tablespoon grated ginger

- Cooked brown rice or quinoa for serving

Preparation:

1. In a bowl, whisk together soy sauce, sesame oil, and cornstarch. Add cubed tofu and toss to coat.

2. Heat vegetable oil in a large skillet or wok over medium-high heat. Add tofu and cook until golden brown on all sides. Remove tofu from skillet and set aside.

3. In the same skillet, add mixed vegetables, garlic, and ginger. Stir-fry until vegetables are tender-crisp.

4. Return tofu to the skillet and toss with vegetables until heated through.

5. Serve stir-fry over cooked brown rice or quinoa.

7. Mediterranean Chickpea Salad

Ingredients:

- 2 cups cooked chickpeas (or 1 can, drained and rinsed)
- 1 cucumber, diced
- 1 cup cherry tomatoes, halved
- 1/4 cup diced red onion
- 1/4 cup chopped fresh parsley
- 2 tablespoons extra virgin olive oil
- 1 tablespoon lemon juice
- 1 teaspoon dried oregano
- Salt and pepper to taste
- Feta cheese for garnish (optional)

Preparation:

1. In a large bowl, combine chickpeas, cucumber, cherry tomatoes, red onion, and parsley.

2. In a small bowl, whisk together olive oil, lemon juice, dried oregano, salt, and pepper.

3. Pour dressing over chickpea mixture and toss to coat.

4. Garnish with crumbled feta cheese, if desired.

5. Serve chilled or at room temperature.

8. Teriyaki Glazed Salmon with Steamed Broccoli

Ingredients:

- 4 salmon fillets

- 1/4 cup low-sodium soy sauce

- 2 tablespoons honey

- 1 tablespoon rice vinegar

- 2 cloves garlic, minced

- 1 teaspoon grated ginger

- 1 tablespoon sesame seeds (optional)

- Steamed broccoli for serving

Preparation:

1. In a small bowl, whisk together soy sauce, honey, rice vinegar, garlic, and ginger to make the teriyaki sauce.

2. Place salmon fillets in a shallow dish and pour teriyaki sauce over them. Let marinate for 15-30 minutes.

3. Preheat oven to 400°F (200°C). Place salmon fillets on a baking sheet lined with parchment paper and bake for 12-15 minutes, or until salmon is cooked through.

4. While salmon is baking, steam broccoli until tender.

5. Serve teriyaki glazed salmon with steamed broccoli, garnished with sesame seeds if desired.

9. Turkey and Vegetable Skewers with Quinoa

Ingredients:

- 1 lb turkey breast, cut into cubes

- 2 bell peppers (any color), cut into chunks

- 1 red onion, cut into chunks

- 1 zucchini, sliced

- 1 tablespoon olive oil

- 1 teaspoon smoked paprika

- 1/2 teaspoon garlic powder

- Salt and pepper to taste

- Cooked quinoa for serving

Preparation:

1. In a bowl, toss turkey cubes and vegetables with olive oil, smoked paprika, garlic powder, salt, and pepper.

2. Thread turkey and vegetable pieces onto skewers, alternating ingredients.

3. Preheat grill or grill pan over medium-high heat. Grill skewers for 10-12 minutes, turning occasionally, until turkey is cooked through and vegetables are tender.

4. Serve turkey and vegetable skewers over cooked quinoa.

10. Ratatouille with Herbed Couscous

Ingredients:

- 1 eggplant, diced

- 2 zucchinis, diced

- 1 bell pepper (any color), diced

- 1 onion, diced

- 2 cloves garlic, minced

- 2 cups diced tomatoes (fresh or canned)

- 1 tablespoon tomato paste

- 1 teaspoon dried thyme

- 1 teaspoon dried basil

- Salt and pepper to taste

- Cooked couscous for serving

Preparation:

1. Heat olive oil in a large skillet or pot over medium heat. Add onion and garlic and cook until softened.

2. Add diced eggplant, zucchini, bell pepper, diced tomatoes, tomato paste, thyme, basil, salt, and pepper to the skillet. Stir to combine.

3. Cover and simmer for 20-25 minutes, stirring occasionally, until vegetables are tender.

4. Meanwhile, prepare couscous according to package instructions.

5. Serve ratatouille over herbed couscous.

Chapter 6

Dishes and Salads

1. Roasted Garlic Mashed Cauliflower

Ingredients:

- 1 head cauliflower, cut into florets

- 3 cloves garlic, minced

- 2 tablespoons olive oil

- Salt and pepper to taste

- 2 tablespoons chopped fresh parsley (optional)

Preparation:

1. Preheat the oven to 400°F (200°C).

2. In a large bowl, toss cauliflower florets and minced garlic with olive oil, salt, and pepper until evenly coated.

3. Spread the cauliflower mixture in a single layer on a baking sheet lined with parchment paper.

4. Roast in the preheated oven for 25-30 minutes, or until cauliflower is tender and golden brown.

5. Transfer the roasted cauliflower to a food processor and pulse until smooth and creamy.

6. Serve hot, garnished with chopped fresh parsley if desired.

2. Quinoa and Black Bean Salad

Ingredients:

- 1 cup cooked quinoa

- 1 can (15 oz) black beans, drained and rinsed

- 1 cup corn kernels (fresh, frozen, or canned)

- 1/4 cup diced red onion

- 1/4 cup chopped fresh cilantro

- Juice of 1 lime

- 2 tablespoons olive oil

- Salt and pepper to taste

Preparation:

1. In a large bowl, combine cooked quinoa, black beans, corn kernels, diced red onion, and chopped cilantro.

2. In a small bowl, whisk together lime juice, olive oil, salt, and pepper.

3. Pour dressing over quinoa mixture and toss to coat.

4. Serve chilled or at room temperature.

3. Steamed Asparagus with Lemon Butter Sauce

Ingredients:

- 1 bunch asparagus, trimmed

- 2 tablespoons butter

- Juice of 1 lemon

- Salt and pepper to taste

Preparation:

1. Steam asparagus in a steamer basket over boiling water for 3-5 minutes, or until crisp-tender.

2. In a small saucepan, melt butter over low heat. Stir in lemon juice, salt, and pepper.

3. Drizzle lemon butter sauce over steamed asparagus before serving.

4. Caprese Salad

Ingredients:

- 2 large tomatoes, sliced

- 1 ball fresh mozzarella cheese, sliced

- Fresh basil leaves

- 2 tablespoons balsamic glaze

- Salt and pepper to taste

Preparation:

1. Arrange tomato slices and mozzarella slices alternately on a serving platter.

2. Tuck fresh basil leaves between tomato and mozzarella slices.

3. Drizzle balsamic glaze over the salad.

4. Season with salt and pepper to taste.

5. Serve immediately as a refreshing side dish.

5. Cucumber Avocado Salad

Ingredients:

- 2 cucumbers, sliced

- 1 avocado, diced

- 1/4 cup diced red onion

- 2 tablespoons chopped fresh dill

- Juice of 1 lemon

- 1 tablespoon olive oil

- Salt and pepper to taste

Preparation:

1. In a large bowl, combine sliced cucumbers, diced avocado, diced red onion, and chopped fresh dill.

2. In a small bowl, whisk together lemon juice, olive oil, salt, and pepper.

3. Pour dressing over cucumber mixture and toss gently to coat.

4. Serve chilled as a light and refreshing salad.

6. Roasted Brussels Sprouts with Balsamic Glaze

Ingredients:

- 1 lb Brussels sprouts, trimmed and halved

- 2 tablespoons olive oil

- Salt and pepper to taste

- 2 tablespoons balsamic glaze

Preparation:

1. Preheat the oven to 400°F (200°C).

2. Toss Brussels sprouts with olive oil, salt, and pepper in a large bowl until evenly coated.

3. Spread Brussels sprouts in a single layer on a baking sheet lined with parchment paper.

4. Roast in the preheated oven for 20-25 minutes, or until Brussels sprouts are caramelized and tender.

5. Drizzle with balsamic glaze before serving.

7. Greek Salad

Ingredients:

- 2 large tomatoes, diced

- 1 cucumber, diced

- 1/2 red onion, thinly sliced

- 1/2 cup Kalamata olives, pitted

- 4 oz feta cheese, crumbled

- 2 tablespoons extra virgin olive oil

- 1 tablespoon red wine vinegar

- 1 teaspoon dried oregano

- Salt and pepper to taste

Preparation:

1. In a large bowl, combine diced tomatoes, diced cucumber, sliced red onion, Kalamata olives, and crumbled feta cheese.

2. In a small bowl, whisk together olive oil, red wine vinegar, dried oregano, salt, and pepper.

3. Pour dressing over salad and toss gently to coat.

4. Serve immediately as a refreshing side dish.

8. Garlic Parmesan Roasted Potatoes

Ingredients:

- 1 1/2 lbs baby potatoes, halved

- 2 tablespoons olive oil

- 2 cloves garlic, minced

- 1/4 cup grated Parmesan cheese

- 1 tablespoon chopped fresh parsley

- Salt and pepper to taste

Preparation:

1. Preheat the oven to 400°F (200°C).

2. In a large bowl, toss halved baby potatoes with olive oil, minced garlic, grated Parmesan cheese, salt, and pepper until evenly coated.

3. Spread potatoes in a single layer on a baking sheet lined with parchment paper.

4. Roast in the preheated oven for 25-30 minutes, or until potatoes are golden brown and crispy.

5. Sprinkle with chopped fresh parsley before serving.

9. Quinoa Tabouli Salad

Ingredients:

- 1 cup cooked quinoa

- 1/2 cucumber, diced

- 1 cup cherry tomatoes, halved

- 1/4 cup chopped fresh parsley

- 2 tablespoons chopped fresh mint

- 2 tablespoons lemon juice

- 1 tablespoon extra virgin olive oil

- Salt and pepper to taste

Preparation:

1. In a large bowl, combine cooked quinoa, diced cucumber, cherry tomatoes, chopped fresh parsley, and chopped fresh mint.

2. In a small bowl, whisk together lemon juice, olive oil, salt, and pepper.

3. Pour dressing over salad and toss gently to coat.

4. Serve chilled or at room temperature.

10. Steamed Green Beans with Almond Gremolata

Ingredients:

- 1 lb green beans, trimmed

- 1/4 cup sliced almonds, toasted

- 2 tablespoons chopped fresh parsley

- 1 tablespoon lemon zest

- 1 clove garlic, minced

- 1 tablespoon extra virgin olive oil

- Salt and pepper to taste

Preparation:

1. Steam green beans in a steamer basket over boiling water for 3-4 minutes, or until crisp-tender.

2. In a small bowl, combine toasted sliced almonds, chopped fresh parsley, lemon zest, minced garlic, olive oil, salt, and pepper to make gremolata.

3. Toss steamed green beans with almond gremolata until evenly coated.

4. Serve hot as a flavorful side dish.

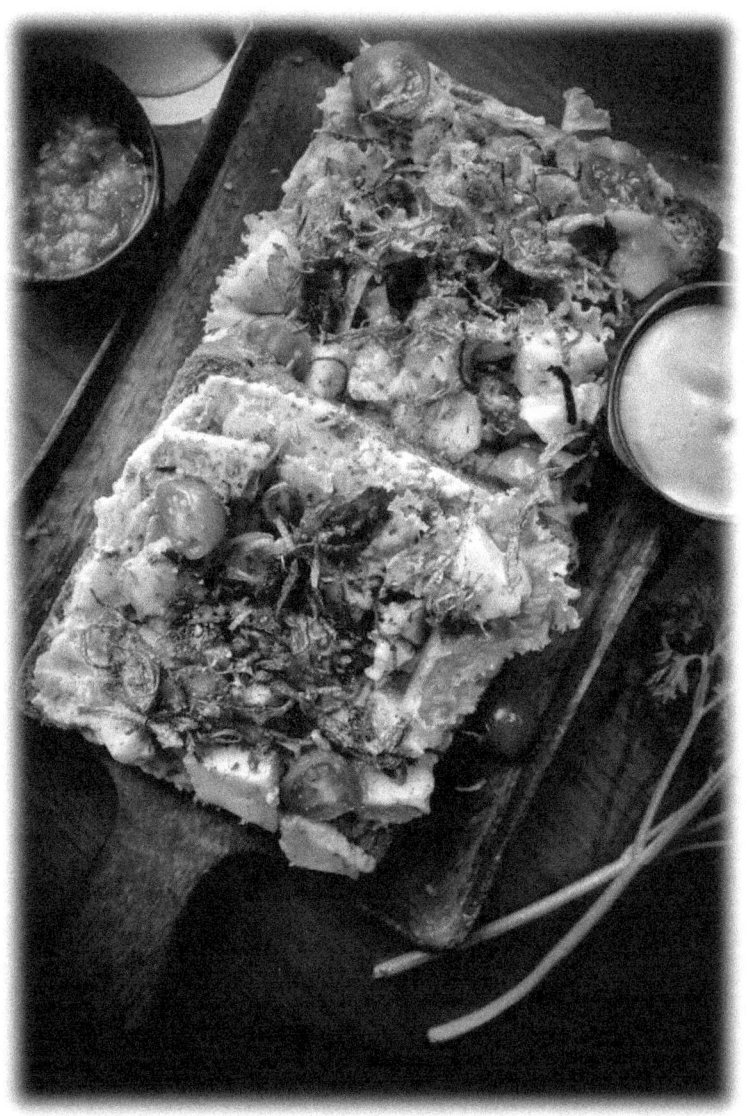

Chapter 7

Desserts and Sweet Treats

These dessert and sweet treat recipes offer a variety of flavors and textures to satisfy your sweet tooth. Enjoy making and indulging in these delicious treats! Adjust ingredients and portions according to your preferences.

These dessert and sweet treat recipes offer a variety of flavors and textures to satisfy your sweet tooth. Enjoy making and indulging in these delicious treats! Adjust ingredients and portions according to your preferences.

1. Berry Parfait

Ingredients:

- 1 cup Greek yogurt

- 1 cup mixed berries (such as strawberries, blueberries, and raspberries)

- 2 tablespoons honey or maple syrup

- 1/4 cup granola

Preparation:

1. In a small bowl, mix Greek yogurt with honey or maple syrup.

2. Layer the yogurt mixture, mixed berries, and granola in serving glasses or bowls.

3. Repeat the layers until the glasses are filled.

4. Serve immediately as a delicious and healthy dessert.

2. Banana Chocolate Chip Oatmeal Cookies

Ingredients:

- 2 ripe bananas, mashed
- 1 cup rolled oats
- 1/4 cup chocolate chips
- 1/4 teaspoon cinnamon
- 1/4 teaspoon vanilla extract

Preparation:

1. Preheat the oven to 350°F (175°C) and line a baking sheet with parchment paper.

2. In a mixing bowl, combine mashed bananas, rolled oats, chocolate chips, cinnamon, and vanilla extract.

3. Drop spoonfuls of the cookie dough onto the prepared baking sheet.

4. Bake in the preheated oven for 12-15 minutes, or until cookies are golden brown.

5. Let cool before serving.

3. Fruit Salad with Honey Lime Dressing

Ingredients:

- 2 cups mixed fruits (such as strawberries, grapes, kiwi, and pineapple), diced

- 2 tablespoons honey

- Juice of 1 lime

- Fresh mint leaves for garnish (optional)

Preparation:

1. In a large bowl, combine diced mixed fruits.

2. In a small bowl, whisk together honey and lime juice to make the dressing.

3. Pour the dressing over the fruit salad and toss gently to coat.

4. Garnish with fresh mint leaves if desired.

5. Serve chilled.

4. Chocolate Avocado Mousse

Ingredients:

- 2 ripe avocados

- 1/4 cup cocoa powder

- 1/4 cup honey or maple syrup

- 1 teaspoon vanilla extract

- Pinch of salt

- Fresh berries for garnish (optional)

Preparation:

1. Scoop the flesh of the avocados into a food processor.

2. Add cocoa powder, honey or maple syrup, vanilla extract, and a pinch of salt.

3. Blend until smooth and creamy, scraping down the sides as needed.

4. Divide the mousse into serving dishes and refrigerate for at least 30 minutes to chill.

5. Garnish with fresh berries before serving.

5. Apple Crisp

Ingredients:

- 4 medium apples, peeled, cored, and sliced

- 1 tablespoon lemon juice

- 1/4 cup granulated sugar

- 1 teaspoon ground cinnamon

- 1/2 cup rolled oats

- 1/4 cup all-purpose flour

- 1/4 cup brown sugar

- 1/4 cup unsalted butter, softened

- Vanilla ice cream for serving (optional)

Preparation:

1. Preheat the oven to 350°F (175°C) and grease a baking dish.

2. In a large bowl, toss sliced apples with lemon juice, granulated sugar, and cinnamon. Transfer to the prepared baking dish.

3. In another bowl, mix rolled oats, all-purpose flour, brown sugar, and softened butter until crumbly.

4. Sprinkle the oat mixture evenly over the apples in the baking dish.

5. Bake in the preheated oven for 30-35 minutes, or until the topping is golden brown and the apples are tender.

6. Serve warm, with vanilla ice cream if desired.

6. Frozen Yogurt Bark

Ingredients:

- 2 cups Greek yogurt

- 2 tablespoons honey or maple syrup

- 1/2 cup mixed berries (such as strawberries, blueberries, and raspberries)

- 2 tablespoons shredded coconut

Preparation:

1. Line a baking sheet with parchment paper.

2. In a bowl, mix Greek yogurt with honey or maple syrup.

3. Spread the yogurt mixture evenly onto the parchment paper.

4. Sprinkle mixed berries and shredded coconut over the yogurt.

5. Place the baking sheet in the freezer for 2-3 hours, or until the yogurt bark is frozen solid.

6. Break the yogurt bark into pieces before serving.

7. Lemon Bars

Ingredients:

- 1 cup all-purpose flour

- 1/2 cup unsalted butter, softened

- 1/4 cup powdered sugar

- 2 large eggs

- 1 cup granulated sugar

- 2 tablespoons all-purpose flour

- 1/4 cup fresh lemon juice

- Zest of 1 lemon

- Powdered sugar for dusting

Preparation:

1. Preheat the oven to 350°F (175°C) and grease a baking dish.

2. In a mixing bowl, combine 1 cup flour, softened butter, and 1/4 cup powdered sugar. Press the mixture into the bottom of the prepared baking dish.

3. Bake the crust in the preheated oven for 15-20 minutes, or until lightly golden.

4. In another bowl, whisk together eggs, granulated sugar, 2 tablespoons flour, lemon juice, and lemon zest until well combined.

5. Pour the lemon mixture over the baked crust and return to the oven. Bake for an additional 20-25 minutes, or until the filling is set.

6. Let cool completely before cutting into bars. Dust with powdered sugar before serving.

8. Grilled Pineapple with Cinnamon Sugar

Ingredients:

- 1 pineapple, peeled, cored, and cut into wedges

- 2 tablespoons brown sugar

- 1 teaspoon ground cinnamon

- Vanilla ice cream for serving (optional)

Preparation:

1. Preheat the grill to medium-high heat.

2. In a small bowl, mix brown sugar and ground cinnamon until well combined.

3. Sprinkle the cinnamon sugar mixture over pineapple wedges, coating them evenly.

4. Grill the pineapple wedges for 2-3 minutes per side, or until grill marks appear and pineapple is heated through.

5. Serve grilled pineapple warm, with a scoop of vanilla ice cream if desired.

9. Chocolate Covered Strawberries

Ingredients:

- 1 cup semisweet chocolate chips

- 1 tablespoon coconut oil

- 12 large strawberries, washed and dried

Preparation:

1. Line a baking sheet with parchment paper.

2. In a microwave-safe bowl, melt semisweet chocolate chips with coconut oil in 30-second intervals, stirring until smooth.

3. Dip each strawberry into the melted chocolate, coating it halfway.

4. Place the chocolate-covered strawberries on the prepared baking sheet.

5. Refrigerate for 15-20 minutes, or until the chocolate is set.

6. Serve chilled.

10. Frozen Banana Pops

Ingredients:

- 2 ripe bananas, peeled and cut in half

- 1/2 cup dark chocolate chips

- 2 tablespoons coconut oil

- Assorted toppings (such as chopped nuts, shredded coconut, or sprinkles)

Preparation:

1. Insert a popsicle stick into each banana half and place them on a parchment-lined baking sheet. Freeze for 1-2 hours, or until firm.

2. In a microwave-safe bowl, melt dark chocolate chips with coconut oil in 30-second intervals, stirring until smooth.

3. Dip each frozen banana pop into the melted chocolate, then immediately sprinkle with your choice of toppings.

4. Place the chocolate-covered banana pops back on the baking sheet and freeze for an additional 30 minutes, or until the chocolate is set.

5. Serve frozen.

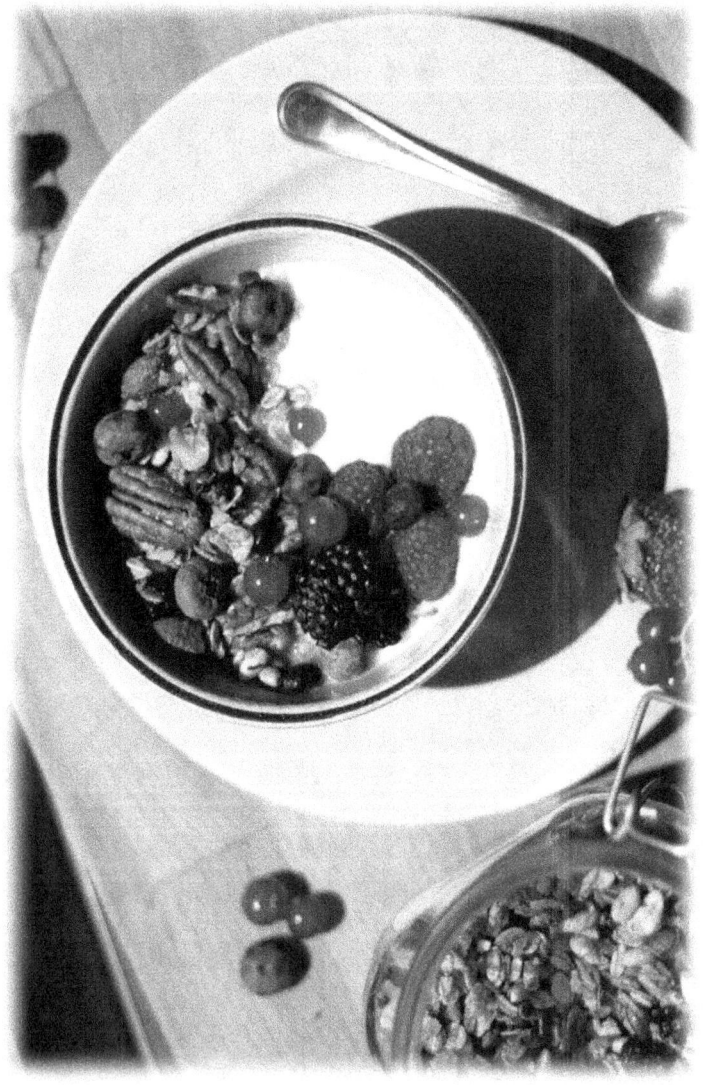

Chapter 8

Refreshing Beverages for Dialysis

These refreshing beverage options are perfect for staying hydrated and enjoying delicious flavors without added sodium or phosphorus. Enjoy them on hot days or anytime you need a refreshing pick-me-up!

1. Infused Water with Cucumber and Mint

Ingredients:

- 1/2 cucumber, sliced

- a handful of fresh mint leaves

- 4 cups water

Preparation:

1. Place cucumber slices and mint leaves in a pitcher.

2. Add water to the pitcher.

3. Refrigerate for at least 1 hour to allow the flavors to infuse.

4. Serve chilled over ice.

2. Hibiscus Iced Tea

Ingredients:

- 2 tablespoons dried hibiscus flowers

- 4 cups water

- 1 tablespoon honey or maple syrup (optional)

- Lemon slices for garnish

Preparation:

1. In a saucepan, bring water to a boil.

2. Add dried hibiscus flowers to the boiling water and remove from heat.

3. Let steep for 10-15 minutes.

4. Strain the tea and discard the hibiscus flowers.

5. Sweeten with honey or maple syrup if desired.

6. Chill in the refrigerator.

7. Serve over ice with lemon slices.

3. Watermelon Lime Cooler

Ingredients:

- 2 cups seedless watermelon, cubed

- Juice of 2 limes

- 2 cups cold water

- Ice cubes

- Fresh mint leaves for garnish (optional)

Preparation:

1. In a blender, puree the watermelon cubes until smooth.

2. Strain the watermelon puree through a fine mesh sieve to remove any pulp.

3. Pour the strained watermelon juice into a pitcher.

4. Add lime juice and cold water to the pitcher and stir to combine.

5. Refrigerate until chilled.

6. Serve over ice with fresh mint leaves for garnish.

4. Ginger Turmeric Golden Milk

Ingredients:

- 2 cups unsweetened almond milk

- 1 teaspoon ground turmeric

- 1/2 teaspoon ground ginger

- 1/4 teaspoon ground cinnamon

- Pinch of black pepper

- 1 tablespoon honey or maple syrup (optional)

Preparation:

1. In a small saucepan, heat almond milk over medium heat.

2. Whisk in turmeric, ginger, cinnamon, and black pepper.

3. Continue to heat until the mixture is hot but not boiling, stirring frequently.

4. Remove from heat and sweeten with honey or maple syrup if desired.

5. Pour into mugs and serve warm.

5. Lemon Ginger Detox Water

Ingredients:

- 4 cups water

- 1 lemon, sliced

- 1-inch piece of ginger, sliced

- Fresh mint leaves

- Ice cubes

Preparation:

1. In a pitcher, combine water, lemon slices, ginger slices, and fresh mint leaves.

2. Refrigerate for at least 1 hour to allow the flavors to infuse.

3. Serve chilled over ice.

6. Green Smoothie

Ingredients:

- 1 cup spinach

- 1/2 cup cucumber, peeled and chopped

- 1/2 cup pineapple chunks

- 1/2 cup unsweetened almond milk

- 1 tablespoon chia seeds

- Ice cubes

Preparation:

1. In a blender, combine spinach, cucumber, pineapple chunks, almond milk, and chia seeds.

2. Blend until smooth.

3. Add ice cubes and blend again until desired consistency is reached.

4. Pour into glasses and serve immediately.

7. Coconut Water Refresher

Ingredients:

- 2 cups coconut water

- 1/4 cup pineapple juice

- Juice of 1 lime

- Ice cubes

- Fresh mint leaves for garnish (optional)

Preparation:

1. In a pitcher, combine coconut water, pineapple juice, and lime juice.

2. Stir well to combine.

3. Chill in the refrigerator.

4. Serve over ice with fresh mint leaves for garnish.

8. Berry Blast Smoothie

Ingredients:

- 1/2 cup mixed berries (such as strawberries, blueberries, and raspberries)

- 1/2 banana

- 1/2 cup unsweetened almond milk

- 1/4 cup Greek yogurt

- 1 tablespoon honey or maple syrup (optional)

- Ice cubes

Preparation:

1. In a blender, combine mixed berries, banana, almond milk, Greek yogurt, and honey or maple syrup.

2. Blend until smooth.

3. Add ice cubes and blend again until desired consistency is reached.

4. Pour into glasses and serve immediately.

9. Minty Lemonade

Ingredients:

- 4 cups water

- Juice of 3 lemons

- 1/4 cup honey or maple syrup

- Handful of fresh mint leaves

- Ice cubes

Preparation:

1. In a pitcher, combine water, lemon juice, honey or maple syrup, and fresh mint leaves.

2. Stir well to dissolve the sweetener.

3. Refrigerate for at least 1 hour to allow the flavors to infuse.

4. Serve chilled over ice.

10. Herbal Tea Blend

Ingredients:

- 1 tablespoon dried nettle leaves

- 1 tablespoon dried dandelion root

- 1 tablespoon dried chamomile flowers

- 4 cups hot water

- Honey or maple syrup to taste (optional)

Preparation:

1. In a teapot, combine dried nettle leaves, dried dandelion root, and dried chamomile flowers.

2. Pour hot water over the herbs.

3. Cover and steep for 10-15 minutes.

4. Strain the tea into cups.

5. Sweeten with honey or maple syrup if desired.

6. Serve warm.

Conclusion

Congratulations on reaching the end of "Kidney Dialysis Diet Cookbook for Women Over 50"! Throughout this book, we've embarked on a journey together to explore the intricacies of managing kidney health through diet and nutrition, specifically tailored for women over the age of 50 undergoing kidney dialysis. As we conclude our exploration, let's reflect on the key insights and takeaways that we've uncovered along the way.

Understanding the importance of nutrition in managing kidney health has been fundamental to our journey. We've delved into the essential role that diet plays in supporting kidney function, while also recognizing the unique dietary considerations that come with undergoing dialysis treatment. By embracing a kidney-friendly diet rich in nutrient-dense foods and mindful of key dietary restrictions, we've empowered ourselves to take proactive steps towards optimizing our health and well-being.

Throughout this book, we've provided comprehensive guidance on navigating the dietary goals and challenges associated with kidney dialysis. From understanding fluid restrictions to identifying key nutrients to focus on, we've equipped ourselves with the knowledge and tools needed to make informed dietary choices that support kidney health. By adopting a balanced and tailored approach to nutrition, we've embraced the opportunity to enhance our overall quality of life and well-being.

Our journey has also been enriched by the diverse array of delicious and nutritious recipes featured in this cookbook. From satisfying breakfast options to nourishing dinners and indulgent desserts, we've explored a variety of culinary creations designed to tantalize the taste buds while adhering to kidney-friendly guidelines. By embracing the abundance of wholesome ingredients and creative cooking techniques at our disposal, we've discovered that eating well can be both enjoyable and nourishing.

In addition to culinary delights, we've also explored a range of refreshing beverages and hydration options ideal for supporting kidney health. From infused waters and herbal teas to nutrient-packed smoothies and revitalizing juices, we've embraced the importance of staying hydrated while savoring flavorful beverages that contribute to our overall well-being.

As we conclude our journey, it's important to recognize that managing kidney health is not just about following a set of dietary guidelines; it's about embracing a holistic approach to self-care that encompasses nutrition, hydration, physical activity, and emotional well-being. By prioritizing self-care and adopting healthy lifestyle habits, we've laid the foundation for long-term health and vitality.

Remember, each step we take towards nourishing our bodies and supporting our kidney health is a testament to our strength, resilience, and commitment to living our best lives. As we move forward, let's continue to embrace the power of nutrition as a cornerstone of our health journey, empowering ourselves to thrive and flourish at every stage of life.

I hope that "Kidney Dialysis Diet Cookbook for Women Over 50" has served as a valuable companion on your path to optimal kidney health and well-being. May the recipes, insights, and guidance shared within these pages continue to inspire and support you on your journey towards a healthier, happier, and more vibrant life.

Wishing you abundance, vitality, and joy on your continued health journey.

Other books by the same author:

1. **Weight Loss Smoothies for Women Over 50**

2. **Kidney Dialysis Diet Cookbook**

3. Smoothies For Diabetes

4. Detoxification and Cleanser Diet for Women

5. Diabetic Renal Diet Cookbook